Pocket G
Radiotherapy
in Clinical Practice

A handbook for first-year students
during clinical placement

Lucy Austin

Lantern

ISBN: 978 1 908625 26 7
Published in 2015 by Lantern Publishing Limited

Lantern Publishing Limited, The Old Hayloft, Vantage Business Park, Bloxham Rd, Banbury
OX16 9UX, UK

www.lanternpublishing.com

British Library Cataloguing in Publication Data
A catalogue record for this book is available from the British Library

The author and publisher have made every attempt to ensure the content of this book
is up to date and accurate. However, healthcare knowledge and information is changing
all the time so the reader is advised to double-check any information in this text on drug
usage, treatment procedures, the use of equipment, etc. to confirm that it complies with the
latest safety recommendations, standards of practice and legislation, as well as local Trust
policies and procedures. Students are advised to check with their tutor and/or mentor before
carrying out any of the procedures in this textbook.

Illustrations by Peter May
Typeset by Medlar Publishing Solutions Pvt Ltd, India
Cover design by Andrew Magee Design Ltd
Printed and bound by 4edge Ltd, Hockley, Essex, UK
Distributed by NBN International, 10 Thornbury Rd, Plymouth PL6 7PP, UK

Personal information

Name: ....

Mobile: ....

Address during placement:...

....

....

....

PLACEMENT DETAILS

Hospital:..

Hospital Address: ....

....

....

....

Number:...

Link lecturer: ....

CONTACT IN CASE OF AN EMERGENCY

Name: ....

Mobile: ....

Home/Work Number:..

Contents

Foreword

The author recently graduated from UWE and this guide is the culmination of her third year dissertation studies. It is hugely refreshing to see a text that has been written by someone in the ideal situation to know exactly what information a new radiotherapy student would find useful. It was only a few years ago that Lucy entered the sometimes daunting area of clinical practice and she has used her own experiences, along with those of her fellow students, to provide the background for this text. This book incorporates some fairly basic concepts along with more complex areas which students often find difficult to master initially.

Lucy genuinely wanted to help her fellow students to understand exactly what it is like to work in a radiotherapy department by providing them with a simple to follow guide in pocket book form. The book has many unique selling points, not least the fairly obvious fact that it is small enough to fit in a uniform pocket, and whilst it contains a wealth of basic information it also provides space for notes so that it is easy to personalise.

We have had many requests for copies of Lucy's book and it will be lovely for Lucy to get the recognition she deserves for all her hard work. As her supervisor it was easy to recognise her passion and talent, but we were thrilled when she also received external recognition in the form of the "Student of the year" award from our professional body, The College of Radiographers, in 2013.

This pocket book will, I am sure, prove to be an invaluable text for students and those new to the radiotherapy environment.

Julie Woodley, PhD, MSc, HDCR, TDCR, FETC
Senior Lecturer, Department of Allied Health Professions,
University of the West of England

Abbreviations

ABC	active breathing control
AP	anteroposterior
ART	adaptive radiotherapy
BCC	basal cell carcinoma
BED	biological effective dose
BEV	beam's eye view
Bx	biopsy
Ca	cancer or carcinoma
CBC	complete blood count
CFRT	conformal radiotherapy
CHART	continuous, hyperfractionated accelerated radiotherapy
CNS	central nervous system
CRT	chemoradiotherapy
CSF	craniospinal fluid
CT	computed tomography
CTV	clinical target volume
d	day
DOB	date of birth
DRR	digital reconstructed radiograph
EBRT	external beam radiotherapy
EPID	electronic portal imaging device
FBC	full blood count
GTV	gross tumour volume
H&H	haemoglobin and haematocrit
HAD	hospital anxiety depression scale
HPV	human papilloma virus
ICC	intercostal catheter

Confusion in the use of abbreviations has been cited as the reason for some clinical incidents. Therefore you should use these abbreviations with caution and only in line with local Trusts' Clinical Governance recommendations which vary between departments!

The correct uniform

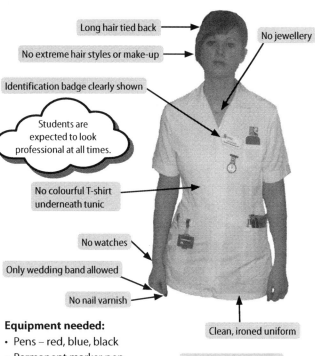

Long hair tied back

No extreme hair styles or make-up

No jewellery

Identification badge clearly shown

Students are expected to look professional at all times.

No colourful T-shirt underneath tunic

No watches

Only wedding band allowed

No nail varnish

Clean, ironed uniform

Shoes should be plain black with toes covered

Equipment needed:

- Pens – red, blue, black
- Permanent marker pen
- Pencil
- 15 cm metal ruler
- Fob watch (optional)
- Notebook (included in this pocket guide)
- Small calculator
- Film card (provided)

YOU are not allowed to work without a **TLD!**

The radiotherapy treatment room

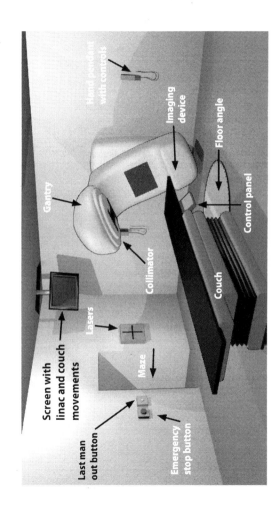

Immobilisation devices

These are some of the immobilisation devices used to stabilise the patient. This is so that they maintain their position throughout treatment. These devices will vary between departments.

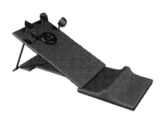

Breast board

This is used to treat the breast. The patient's head lies in the doughnut-shaped pad and the arms are raised into the cup-shaped holders. Either one or both arms are raised, depending on the department and technique.

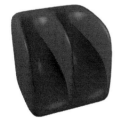

Ankle/foot support

This is used to stabilise the patient's feet, and is typically used on prostate and bladder treatments.

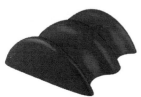

Knee support

This is used to help the patient maintain their position by supporting their knees and back; this pad is used on most treatments.

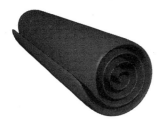

Camping mat

Typically used for patients lying prone, or palliative patients who may struggle to lie on the hard carbon fibre treatment bed.

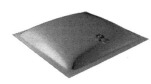

Vac bag

This reusable bag contains lots of small polystyrene balls which are moulded around the patient. A vacuum pump then sucks all of the air out, making it firm, and an imprint is then made of the patient. This can then be used for each fraction.

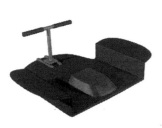

Wing board

This is used to treat the chest. The patient holds the T-bar or a U-shaped bar whilst their head lies on the head pad. Sometimes a Vac bag is placed inside this for additional support. The patient's elbows rest on the wings of the board.

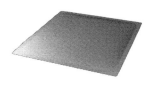

Bolus

This is typically used on breast techniques; it is placed over the patient's skin and secured using tape. Bolus is used to bring the isodose up to the skin surface. The material is tissue equivalent to the skin density.

Wax

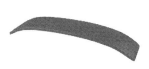

This can be used to create a uniform block. It is placed or shaped around the treatment area, for example the nose for electron treatments. This makes the dose distribution more homogeneous.

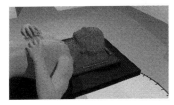

Head mask

Head masks are individually shaped for each patient. The sides of the mask are moulded around the face and secured using either clips or blocks. Claustrophobic patients can struggle greatly with this device, and sometimes a bite block is required to immobilise the tongue and nose plugs. The mask can extend to below the shoulders. This device is used on patients with head/neck cancers.

Hospital bins

Hospitals have colour-coded bins to determine what type of waste should be put in them.
It is important that you dispose of any waste in the appropriate bin.

Colour of bin	Use	Example
Black	Domestic waste	Packaging
Yellow	Hazardous and infectious waste	Gloves, aprons, items with blood on
Yellow with black line	Offensive waste	Incontinence pads
Purple	Cytotoxic waste	Chemotherapy drugs
Orange	Infectious waste	Dressings

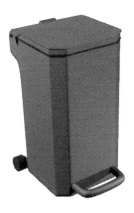

Any paper containing patient information needs to be shredded separately. There is a separate bin/bag for this.

Top tips

1. First impressions last, so it's important to be professional and punctual at all times.

2. If you are required to undertake any research or paperwork during your placement, ensure you begin it as soon as possible to allow for checking and alterations by a practice educator.

3. Always ask if you don't understand or if you are unsure about what is happening – you are there to learn.

4. Think about any desirable experiences as soon as possible, so you can get them organised quicker, and make the most of your time available in the department.

5. You may be expected to do mental arithmetic on the treatment floor. If you struggle with this you may want to practise beforehand or use a pocket calculator.

6. Be comfortable saying to a patient *"Sorry, I am a student, let me just ask/get my colleague"*.

7. Try to have a walk around the department and familiarise yourself. The quicker you know your way around, the easier it is to settle.

Sharps bin

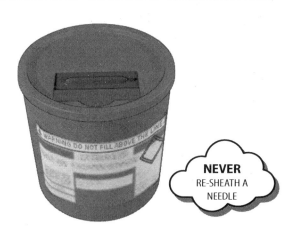

NEVER RE-SHEATH A NEEDLE

ANY sharp instruments must be placed in a yellow/orange 'sharps bin' after use, for incineration.

Remember to partially close the lid after each use but do not fully close the lid as it will permanently lock. Only fully close the bin when it is filled to the max line, to avoid a costly wastage of materials.

When using sharp materials such as a needle you should have a sharps bin within reach in order to dispose of the instrument immediately.

Do not leave any sharp materials for someone else to clear.

Do not walk around with a needle or sharp instrument. If you need to put the needle down, simply dispose of it and use a new one.

Do not use any sterilized equipment which is already opened – you do not know if it has already been used!

How to make a permanent skin mark (tattoo)

Not all students will be able to tattoo the patient in their first year, but if you do here are some helpful tips. Remember, only undertake this procedure if you feel confident and fully understand the process.

- Stay calm at all times; this will help the patient stay relaxed.
- Take your time! You should not feel as if you need to be rushed.
- Ensure you are supervised, as a qualified member of staff needs to sign that the tattoo has been completed successfully.
- Ensure you have everything you need BEFORE you start.
- Check the patient has consented to having the tattoo and explain the procedure.
- Bring tray/trolley with equipment to the patient.
- Wipe the skin clean with an antibacterial wipe.
- DO NOT use an already opened/unsheathed needle.
- Wear gloves/apron AND wash hands before and after.
- Pierce the skin at an 45° angle, then lift slightly to allow the ink to flow under the skin.
- Either syringe ink into the needle beforehand or dab ink onto the pierced skin using a new cotton bud.
- Place needle immediately into sharps bin once finished. If needle needs to be put down, bin it, and use a new one.
- Wipe excess ink from skin, check the tattoo has been clearly made and dispose of equipment using appropriate bins.
- Procedures and protocols may vary between centres. You should read the local guidance before undertaking any permanent skin mark-up.

Take time to listen to your patient!

Do not use medical language which will confuse the patient.

Patients may be very anxious; talk in a calm manner at all times.

Be aware of who can over hear your conversation with the patient.

Effective Communication

Appear welcoming and approachable.

Maintain eye contact which is comfortable for you and your patient.

Body language is important when engaging your patient – hand gestures can help illustrate a point.

It is important to look interested in what the patient is saying to you.

Reference: Easton, S. (2008) *An Introduction to Radiography.* London: Churchill Livingstone, pp 23–40.

First day chat

Six key points to remember when treating the patient for the first time:

1. Check the patient has signed the consent form and still consents to treatment. A pregnancy form must be completed by all females aged 10–55 years. This must be done BEFORE the patient starts their treatment.

2. Identify the patient using 3 forms of positive identification:
   - Full name, first line of address and area being treated.

3. Make sure the patient understands any side-effects they may experience and explain that these will not happen immediately. It is usually at least a week before they may start to notice any changes.

4. Ask the patient if they have any questions or concerns before they start treatment. Explain any terminology the patient may not be familiar with on their appointment list, such as machine name and what the review appointments are. It would be good to mention that the patient will not see or feel anything during the treatment.

5. Run through what the patient will expect during their treatment. For example, diodes being stuck onto the patient and the noises the machine makes.

6. Explain that the radiographers can still see and hear the patient at all times so we can stop the machine immediately if there is a problem.

A relaxed patient will set up more quickly and smoothly

Couch moves

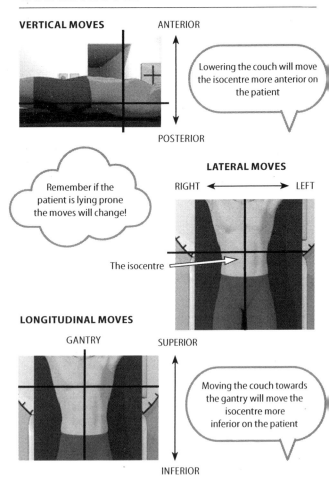

VERTICAL MOVES

ANTERIOR

Lowering the couch will move the isocentre more anterior on the patient

POSTERIOR

Remember if the patient is lying prone the moves will change!

LATERAL MOVES

RIGHT ←→ LEFT

The isocentre ⇦

LONGITUDINAL MOVES

GANTRY

SUPERIOR

Moving the couch towards the gantry will move the isocentre more inferior on the patient

INFERIOR

Isocentre calculations

Once a patient has been lined up to the tattoos, there may be some alterations to the couch. This is to move the planning target volume to the isocentre.

This does not apply for all patient set-ups.

Move to be made	Couch orientation
Superior 'Sup'	**Subtract:** from the <u>longitudinal</u> value
Inferior 'Inf'	**Add:** on to the <u>longitudinal</u> value
Posterior 'Post'	**Subtract:** from the <u>vertical</u> value
Anterior 'Ant'	**Add:** on to <u>vertical</u> value
Left	**Subtract:** from the <u>lateral</u> value
Right	**Add:** on to the <u>lateral</u> value

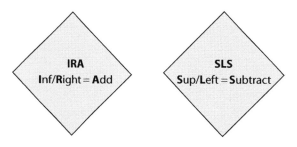

IRA
Inf/Right = Add

SLS
Sup/Left = Subtract

Laser positioning

The position of the lasers in relation to the tattoo is often stated throughout the set-up process. We are aiming to get the tattoo in the centre of the cross (isocentre) on both sides of the patient.

Below is a step-by-step process of understanding what is being stated.

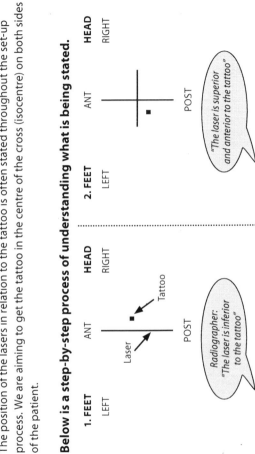

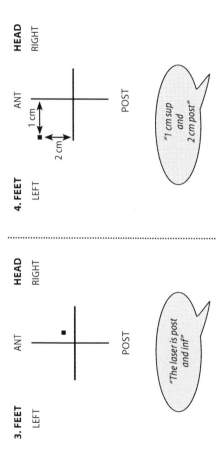

3. FEET — LEFT   ANT   **HEAD** — RIGHT   POST

"The laser is post and inf"

4. FEET — LEFT   ANT   **HEAD** — RIGHT   POST

1 cm   2 cm

"1 cm sup and 2 cm post"

This explains where the laser is in relation to the tattoo. In some departments this could be the other way around; for example, the position of the tattoo could be described in relation to where the laser is. You should clarify this when you first start working on the treatment unit, to avoid confusion.

Before setting up the patient

Before we start aligning the tattoos with the lasers, there are a few things to remember.

- Has the first day chat been undertaken, if it is the patient's first treatment? (see page 11).
- Have you correctly identified your patient? i.e. date of birth and name (first line of address is done on the first day).
- Have you asked how the patient is today? They may be worried about something or have some questions. It is important to check with your patient that they are not struggling with any side-effects that we can help with.
- Have you reminded the patient that they need to wait after treatment to see the doctor/review radiographer? (if applicable).
- Has the patient removed the item(s) of clothing required for the treatment area before getting onto the couch?
- Once the patient is lying on the bed you should check that they are lying straight. This is done by making sure the sagittal laser (laser going down the length of the couch) is running through the middle of the sternum. Standing at the end of the couch will also help you to see if the patient is straight.

Once you have done this, the next step will be aligning the tattoos with the lasers.
Having the patient straight to start with will make this process a lot easier!

How to align the tattoos

Before any shifts can be done, the two lateral tattoos (the tattoos on the patient's sides) need to be level. In order to do this we move the bed so the isocentre is on one of the lateral tattoos (the isocentre is where the lasers make a cross). Now one tattoo is aligned, we need to move the patient so both lateral tattoos are in the centre of the cross (isocentre). Here are some tips on how we can manipulate the patient in order to get the tattoos level with each other.

Chest rotation

In this example we want to move the tattoo more anterior. To do this, try placing your hands on either side of the patient's chest and moving the right side down and the left side up. Rotating the patient this way will make the tattoo on the opposite side more posterior so the radiographer will raise the bed.

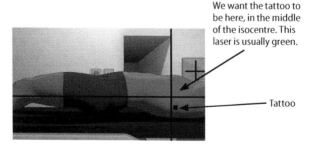

We want the tattoo to be here, in the middle of the isocentre. This laser is usually green.

Tattoo

Breast alignment

This technique takes time and practice. To move the tattoo more superior, try placing your hand on the inside of the patient's upper arm and raise the elbow slightly, ensuring that the patient's skin does not stick to the bed. This should make the tattoo more superior. The opposite will move the tattoo more inferior.

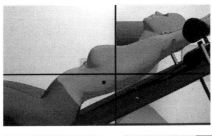

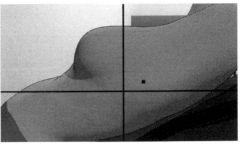

As you can see in the picture above, if the patient's tattoo is very superior (in relation to the lasers), the patient may be tense and so be holding their position – try to get them to relax.

Pelvis alignment

For 'ant' and 'post' movements rotate the patient's hips in a similar method to that you would use for the chest rotations. If your tattoo is superior you can move the patient's leg for minor changes, or ask the patient to stretch down his/her leg for large movements. If the tattoo is very inferior, ask the patient to stretch down with the opposite leg.

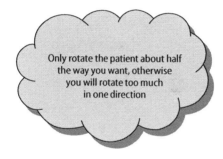

Only rotate the patient about half the way you want, otherwise you will rotate too much in one direction

See page 13 for explanations on the direction of movement for the terminology above.

Naming different beam angles

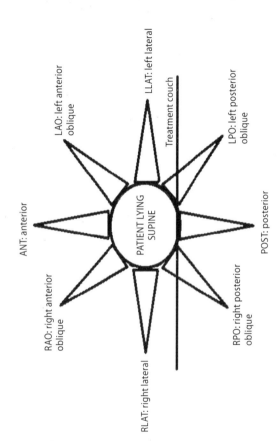

ANT: anterior

LAO: left anterior oblique

LLAT: left lateral

Treatment couch

LPO: left posterior oblique

POST: posterior

RPO: right posterior oblique

RLAT: right lateral

RAO: right anterior oblique

PATIENT LYING SUPINE

How can cancer spread?

When a cancer spreads away from the primary cancer it is known to be 'metastatic' and the secondary cancer that forms is called a 'metastasis' or 'metastases' for more than one. There are 5 main routes of spread:

Blood stream
Usually sarcomas. A cancer cell can get stuck in the thin-walled capillary and grow.

Direct invasion
Where the cancer invades neighbouring tissues.

Lymphatic system
Carcinomas usually spread through the lymphatic system to local lymph nodes first. For example, breast cancer can spread to axillary lymph nodes.

Implantation
Where the cancer is spread through medical instruments or naturally. For example, during surgery some cells may be left in the scar tissue or along the ureters to the bladder.

Transcoelomic
Spread across body cavities, this can happen during surgery or direct invasion.

Typical radiotherapy techniques

Radical prostate
Techniques will vary between departments

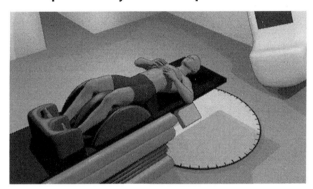

Typical beam arrangement

IMRT or three beams: one anterior beam and two lateral (oblique) beams. The lateral beams are wedged to conform to the curvature of the patient's surface.

Patient position

Supine, head to gantry, hands on chest. Organ motion can be controlled by bladder or rectum preparation prior to each treatment.

Immobilisation devices

Stocks or Vac bag to secure the patient's feet, along with a knee support.

Typical prescription

64–70 Gy, in 32–35# with 2 Gy/# (fraction), over 7 weeks.

Radical breast

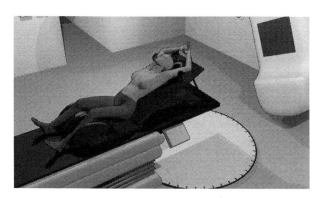

Typical beam arrangement

Two beams in a tangential field pair arrangement.

Patient position

Patient is supine and sitting up slightly on the angled breast board with one or both arms up. Knees are slightly bent. Some departments provide special breast gowns to maintain patient dignity.

Immobilisation devices

A breast board with attachable head support and arm rests. A knee support helps prevent the patient from sliding down the board.

Typical prescriptions

50 Gy in 25# with 2 Gy/# over 5 weeks.

40 Gy in 15# with 2 Gy/# over 3 weeks.

Breast boards can get very cold. Putting a pillowcase on the board can help with this.

Radical bladder

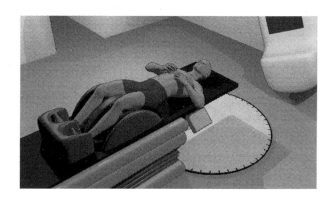

Beam arrangement

Three beams: one anterior and two posterior oblique beams.

Patient position

Supine, head to gantry, hands on chest.

Immobilisation devices

Stocks or Vac bag to secure the patient's feet. Head pads could be used to reduce movement of the head.

Typical prescriptions

64 Gy in 32# with 2 Gy/# over 6.5 weeks.

55 Gy in 20# with 2 Gy/# over 4 weeks.

Radiographers need to check if the patient has undertaken their bladder or rectal preparations.

Radical lung

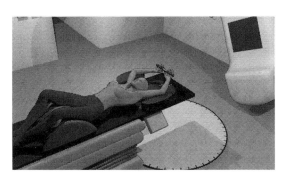

Beam arrangement

This arrangement varies greatly depending on the tumour location. A three-field beam arrangement is usually used, with varying oblique and lateral angles.

Patient position

Supine, both arms raised above head holding onto the bar, elbows resting on the wings of the board. Knees slightly bent.

Immobilisation devices

A wing board is used with a T-bar attached; this is adjustable for each patient. A Vac bag may be used for additional support around the chest with a knee support. Only clothing from the waist up needs to be removed.

Typical prescriptions

NSCLC – 55 Gy in 20# over 4 weeks.

      66 Gy in 33# over 6.5 weeks.

SCLC – 40 Gy in 15# over 3 weeks.

Radical rectum

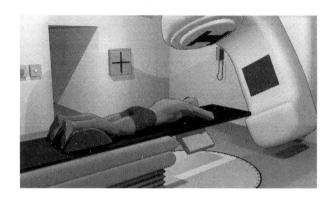

Beam arrangement

Three beams: 1 posterior and two wedged lateral fields.

Patient position

Prone, heels apart, head resting on hands.

Immobilisation devices

Knee support or Vac bag to secure feet. A camping mat for additional comfort is sometimes used.

Typical prescription

45–50 Gy in 25# with 2 Gy/# over 5 weeks.

References: Hanna, L ., Crosby, T. and Macbeth, F. (2008) *Practical Clinical Oncology*. Cambridge: Cambridge University Press. Barrett, A *et al*. (2009) *Practical Radiotherapy Planning*. 4th ed. London. Taylor & Francis.

Tolerance doses

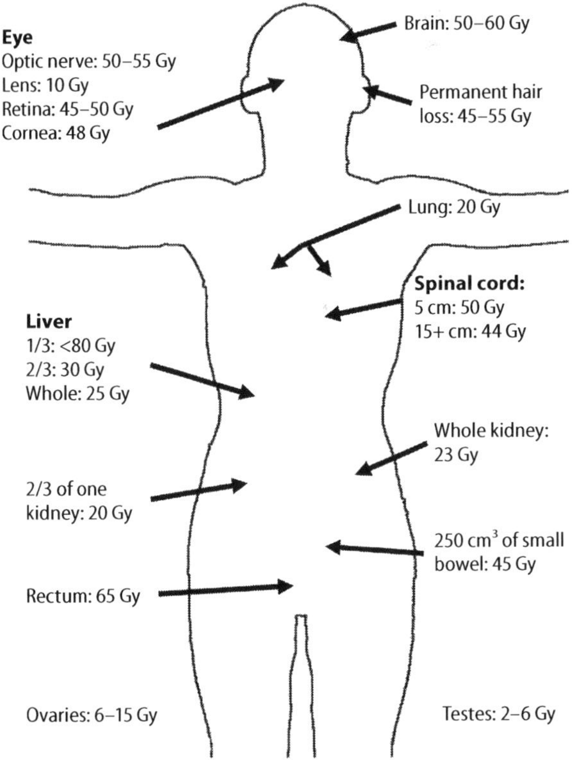

Eye
Optic nerve: 50–55 Gy
Lens: 10 Gy
Retina: 45–50 Gy
Cornea: 48 Gy

Brain: 50–60 Gy

Permanent hair loss: 45–55 Gy

Lung: 20 Gy

Spinal cord:
5 cm: 50 Gy
15+ cm: 44 Gy

Liver
1/3: <80 Gy
2/3: 30 Gy
Whole: 25 Gy

Whole kidney: 23 Gy

2/3 of one kidney: 20 Gy

250 cm³ of small bowel: 45 Gy

Rectum: 65 Gy

Ovaries: 6–15 Gy

Testes: 2–6 Gy

Reference: Barrett, A et al. (2009) *Practical Radiotherapy Planning*. 4th ed. London: Taylor & Francis, pp. 46–51.

What is...Brachytherapy?

- 'Brachy' means 'short' in Greek so it is 'short therapy'.
- The radioactive substances are placed **directly into** or **very close** to the tumour.
- Radioactive materials or 'sources' include seeds, tubes and needles.
- The implant **can be left** for a period of time or permanently.
- A **higher dose** can be given to a **smaller area** compared with radiotherapy.
- Dose is given off **continuously**.
- The most common treatment you will come across using brachytherapy is for **prostate** cancer for men and **gynaecological** cancers in women.

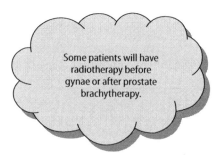

Some patients will have radiotherapy before gynae or after prostate brachytherapy.

Reference: CancerHelp UK (2011) *Cancer Treatments*. Available at: http://cancerhelp.cancerresearchuk.org/about-cancer/treatment/radiotherapy/internal/

What is...Electron treatment?

- Electrons are used for **superficial** treatments.
- This can include skin cancers or a '**boost**' to scar tissues.
- Very **minimal** side-effects, usually only erythema.
- This treatment does not usually have pre-planned gantry/collimator angles; skin apposition is used to set up the patient.
- Electrons **diverge** more than photons, which is why the applicator is so close to the patient's skin.
- The '**effective treatment depth**' in cm is approximately 1/3 of the beam energy in MeV, e.g. 9 MeV treats to the effective depth of 3 cm.
- Different tissue densities, e.g. air and cartilage, can cause non-homogeneous (uneven) dose distributions.

When setting up the patient, an even skin apposition needs to be achieved (*see* pp. 30–31). A lead cut-out is placed into the applicator rather than placed on the patient for electron treatments.

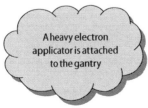

A heavy electron applicator is attached to the gantry

Reference: Barrett, A *et al.* (2009) *Practical Radiotherapy Planning*. 4th ed. London: Taylor & Francis, p. 21.

What is...Orthovoltage and superficial X-ray therapy?

- Used for areas on/close to the **skin surface**, such as skin cancers.

- Orthovoltage uses a **higher energy** kilovoltage, whereas SXR (superficial X-ray) uses a **lower energy** kilovoltage treatment.

- The X-ray energy varies: up to 200 kV (kilovolts) for SXR and up to 500 kV for orthovoltage.

- It is not essential for the patient to lie on a hard carbon fibre bed. Instead they can sit or lie on a hospital bed, which makes this treatment more **comfortable**.

- The field shape and size is created by an **applicator** and a **lead cut-out**. A doctor will choose which shape and size to use during the planning stage.

- Lead shapes are also used for **extra shielding and immobilisation** of sensitive tissues, such as eyes. Lead stops the X-rays from penetrating the healthy skin.

- Immobilisation devices such as Vac bags (*see* pp. 3–5) may be required for most patients, as the time to deliver treatment can be long. Typically this treatment is used on elderly patients who may find it harder to maintain their position throughout the treatment.

- This treatment is a '**free set-up**' so there are no set collimator or gantry angles. The radiographer will set the applicator so the distance between the applicator and the skin surface is as even as possible. This is known as '**skin apposition**'.

- Due to the size and shape of some cancers an even skin apposition can be difficult to achieve; there may be '**stand off**' or '**stand in**'.
- This set-up is similar for electron treatments. The main difference in set-up with electrons is that lasers and the FSD are used to achieve the correct distance between the applicator and skin.

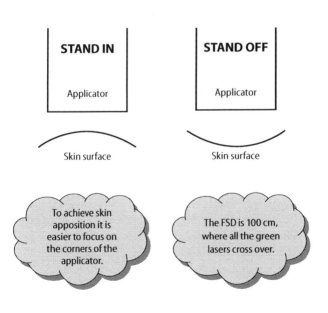

STAND IN

Applicator

Skin surface

STAND OFF

Applicator

Skin surface

To achieve skin apposition it is easier to focus on the corners of the applicator.

The FSD is 100 cm, where all the green lasers cross over.

What is...IGRT?

- IGRT stands for Image Guided Radiotherapy.
- IGRT is where the imaging is used to **increase the accuracy of treatment by reducing positional errors that can occur**.
- An image is taken on the treatment set and is **compared** with the image created when the patient was initially planned.
- Most departments will have different imaging protocols for each treatment site. A 'typical' imaging protocol for a radical patient could be:
  - imaging every day for the first 3 days
  - then undertake a systematic analysis
  - if no moves are required, imaging is required once a week.
- Imaging can be '**online**' or '**offline**'. Online is when the images are being checked just before the patient has their treatment, whilst offline is when a radiographer checks the images after the patient has had their treatment.
- Online imaging allows the radiographer to make small **adjustments** to the treatment couch before delivering the treatment. This will be only a matter of a few millimetres but will make it more accurate and is known by radiographers as '**doing a move**'.
- **At least two** members of staff should check the images taken, and one radiographer should be a senior.

- Each cancer site will have a margin where the image is:
  In tolerance: the image matches the reference image enough to ensure accurate treatment.
  Out of tolerance: the image is not a close match to the reference image, and more imaging may be required in the next fraction. The moves made when setting up the patient may be altered slightly and checked with more imaging.
  Gross error: It is not safe to treat because the patient's position is out of the safe margin to treat.
- After a few images a **statistical analysis** is undertaken, where an average and standard deviation is calculated. The average value is the move required for a 'perfect match'; for example, the patient needs to be 4 mm to the left to be in the exact anatomical position in comparison to when they were planned.
- The RCR (2008) have many guidelines on imaging and how it should be used within the department.

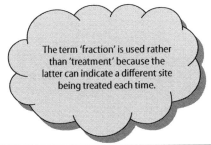

The term 'fraction' is used rather than 'treatment' because the latter can indicate a different site being treated each time.

Reference: The Royal College of Radiologists, Society and College of Radiographers, Institute of Physics and Engineering in Medicine (2008) *On Target: ensuring geometric accuracy in radiotherapy*. London: The College of Radiologists, p. 26.

What is...IMRT?

- IMRT stands for Intensity Modulated Radiotherapy.

- This is a technique used mostly on radical prostate, breast, and head and neck cancers.

- IMRT techniques alter the **intensity of the beam**, providing a **better dose distribution and tumour coverage** than conventional radiotherapy.

- The shape of the beam can be changed through the MLC (multi-leaf collimator). The MLC can move **continuously** while the treatment beam is being delivered, in either multiple beams or one continuous beam where the gantry rotates all around the patient.

- IMRT allows for **dose escalation** to the tumour whilst also sparing sensitive structures such as the spinal cord.

- Increasing the dose to the cancer increases the **TCP** (tumour control probability) and so the **prognosis of the patient improves**.

- A reduced dose to normal tissues will result in fewer side-effects both in the short and long term. This improves the overall quality of life for the patient.

- Some IMRT treatments are quicker than conventional radiotherapy, especially if one continuous beam is used rather than multiple beams. The patient is thus on the treatment couch for less time, which gives a better patient experience than conventional radiotherapy.

What is...Hormone therapy?

Some patients may be put on hormone therapy. This treatment can be used to shrink or control tumours or reduce the risk of cancer returning. This is mostly used for breast and prostate cancers.

The main aims of hormone therapy are to lower oestrogen/ testosterone levels or to block the receptors on the cancerous cell in order to starve it of the oestrogen/ testosterone which encourages tumour growth.

Not all patients are able to have this treatment because it depends on the receptors present on the cells' surface.

The following is a list of some hormone therapy drugs used:

Brand name	Generic name	Application
Arimidex	Anastrozole	To treat breast cancer An aromatase inhibitor For post-menopausal women One tablet a day
Aromasin	Exemestane	To treat breast cancer For post-menopausal women An aromatase inhibitor One tablet a day
Casodex	Bicalutamide	To treat prostate cancer Injection or oral every 28 days
Zoladex	Goserelin	To treat breast and prostate cancer Injection, for 2 years For pre-menopausal women
Tamoxifen	Novadex	To treat breast cancer 20 mg Anti-oestrogen drug Adjuvant therapy taken for 5 years

What is...Chemotherapy?

- Chemotherapy is a **systemic** treatment using a **cytotoxic** drug which involves the whole body.
- Chemotherapy may be one or a variety of drugs combined in a regime and 'cycles'.
- It can be administered either **intravenously, orally or topically**.
- Cancerous cells are continuously dividing by **mitosis**. Chemotherapy drugs **damage the cell's genes** when the cell is dividing, causing the cell to die.
- It can be used:
  - **to treat** any potential metastatic spread
  - **to shrink** the tumour for surgery or radiotherapy
  - as a sole **curative** treatment.
- **Chemoradiotherapy** is when chemotherapy is used at the same time as radiotherapy. The drugs make the cells more radiosensitive.
- Not all cancers are **sensitive** to chemotherapy.
- Patients with chemotherapy will experience **additional** side-effects. You should know what these are, so you can **differentiate** between chemotherapy and radiotherapy side-effects.

> Side-effects are caused by damage to normal cells; this is true for all treatments.

Reference: Cancer Help UK (2011) *Cancer Treatments*. Available at: http://cancerhelp.cancerresearchuk.org/about-cancer/treatment/chemotherapy/

Chemotherapy side-effects

As with radiotherapy, individual patients will experience varying severity of side-effects. Each drug will have its own list of specific side-effects, and the patient will be made aware of these before they are asked for consent for treatment. The following are general side-effects of chemotherapy.

Side-effect	Details
Anaemia	Low red blood count, causing tiredness and fatigue.
Hair loss	Hair follicles have a high cell turnover and are rapidly growing, so are targeted by the drug. Hair loss is reversible.
Neutropenia	Low neutrophil cell count, weakened immune system, increased risk of infection.
Nausea and vomiting	Steroids are usually given to help with nausea and to support appetite.
Diarrhoea	This can be made worse by radiotherapy if treating the pelvic region.
Dermatological toxicity	Some drugs can enhance reactions from radiotherapy such as cisplatin.
Altered sense of taste	Some patients notice a metallic taste in their mouth or total loss of the sense of taste.
Mucositis	Oral mucositis results from use of some chemotherapy drugs, because of the high cell turnover the drugs target.

Most chemotherapy side-effects will fade away once treatment has stopped.

Radiotherapy side-effects

Skin reactions

Side-effects	Advice and medication
Erythema (mild reaction)	• Ensure the patient is not using any soaps/ perfumes/ deodorants which may contain metallic components. • Patients are advised to only use 'Simple' soap. • Moisturise twice a day with aqueous cream. Putting the cream in the fridge may help reduce the hot feeling. • Check the skin has not broken. • Loose fitting clothing can reduce friction.
Dry desquamation (moderate reaction)	• Ensure that the patient is following the advice indicated above. • Fucibet (antibiotic cream) can be provided, to prevent infection. • If the patient has pruritus, 1% hydrocortisone can be prescribed. This should be given up to four times a day.
Moist desquamation (severe reaction)	• The patient must stop using the aqueous cream, and a dressing may be needed. • Hydrogel, which acts like another layer of skin, may be required. • Check with a swab to ensure the area is not infected.

See page 52 for a glossary on medical terminology.

> Skin reactions are worse in areas where skin folds cause friction, for example, under the breast.

Brain and central nervous system

Side-effects	Advice and medication
• Raised intracranial pressure causing headaches, nausea, blurred vision and an unsteady gait • Tiredness • Dysphasia • Hair loss	• Ensure the patient is drinking plenty of fluids • Dexamethasone: a steroid which can be prescribed to reduce the intra-cranial pressure • Maxalon: an antiemetic for nausea

Neck and thorax

Side-effects	Advice and medication
• Pain • Dysphagia • Mucositis • Xerostomia • Weight loss • Hair loss • Fungal infection • Haemoptysis • Breathlessness	• Refer patient to the dietician and speech and language therapist if problems persist. Nutritional drinks can be provided in order to reduce the weight loss. • Analgesics such as paracetamol and oromorph are provided to help the patient swallow soft food more easily. • General advice such as avoiding alcohol and spicy foods and stopping smoking will help reduce side-effects. • Nystatin: prevents any fungal infection. • Difflam: treats mucositis. • Artificial saliva: for xerostomia. • Antacid: helps with dysphagia.

Breast

Side-effects	Advice and medication
• Pain • Tiredness • Severe skin reaction	• Skin reaction can be worse due to friction. It should be suggested that the patient wears a non-wired bra with loose fitting clothing, whilst still following the skin care advice. • Analgesics such as paracetamol can be provided to reduce the pain/heaviness.

Pelvic region

Side-effects	Advice and medication
• Difficulty in micturation • Cystitis • Haematuria • Proctitis • Diarrhoea • Tiredness	• A mid-stream urine (MSU) sample should be taken to ensure the cystitis is radiation induced and not due to infection. Cranberry juice is often suggested to those patients who are NOT on medication for a heart problem. Increased fluid intake will also reduce discomfort. • Information on appropriate diet should be given, including advice on eating less fibre. • The patient may be taking milk of magnesia in order to have an empty bowel for treatment. If so, reduce the amount being taken. • Loperamide: relieves diarrhoea if dietary changes fail.

Reference: Watson *et al.* (2006) *Oncology*. 2nd ed. Oxford: Oxford University Press, pp. 59–60.

Blood values

Some patients will undergo a weekly blood test to ensure that they are not anaemic, as this will affect the effectiveness of radiotherapy. Anaemia is when the patient's haemoglobin levels are low; haemoglobin in red blood cells carries the oxygen, and when there is less haemoglobin and therefore less oxygen in the body, cells can be hypoxic. Hypoxic cells are radio-resistant, therefore radiotherapy is not as effective. If the haemoglobin level becomes too low a blood transfusion may be required. A blood test can also monitor the white blood count as this can indicate if the patient is immunosuppressed or has a possible infection.

Haematology	Male	Female
White blood cell (WBC)	$4–11 \times 10^9$/L	$4–11 \times 10^9$/L
Red blood cell (RBC)	$4.5–6.5 \times 10^{12}$/L	$3.8–5 \times 10^{12}$/L
Haemoglobin (Hb)	13–18 g/mL	12–16 g/mL
Neutrophil	$2.0–7.5 \times 10^9$/L	$2.0–7.5 \times 10^9$/L
Platelets (thrombocytes)	$150–440 \times 10^9$/L	$150–440 \times 10^9$/L

References: Longmore, M *et al.* (2014) *Oxford Handbook of Clinical Medicine.* Oxford: Oxford University Press. Waugh, A. & Grant, A. *Ross and Wilson: Anatomy and Physiology in Health and Illness.* Churchill Livingstone. 9th ed. Both cited in Cancer Research UK (2013) at www.cancerresearchuk.org/cancer-help/about-cancer/cancer-questions/what-is-a-normal-full-blood-count

Patient advice

Another test which may be required during radiotherapy if a patient suffers from cystitis is a mid-stream urine sample (MSU). This is to ensure that the cystitis is a radiation-induced side-effect and not due to an infection which would require antibiotics.

As a health care professional it is important when giving any advice or medication that the patient fully understands any instructions given. It may be useful to write down any important information and most departments have information leaflets which are available for patients.

The side-effects experienced will vary between patients; some patients will have more severe side-effects than others even though they have had the same treatment.

Other rarer side-effects can occur with radiotherapy treatment, such as pneumonitis, cerebral oedema, somnolence syndrome and pulmonary embolism.

Always try to first advise patients on how to change their lifestyle or diet to help relieve radiotherapy side-effects, as it is not always necessary to give medication.

Radiographers can refer patients to other health care professionals such as dieticians, if the patient is losing weight, or a speech and language therapist. Most patients having treatment to the head and neck will require this additional support and close monitoring of their weight.

If you are unsure on how to advise a patient on a particular side-effect always speak with another health care professional for support.

Patients undergoing radiotherapy to the abdomen can suffer from nausea and vomiting; this is because radiotherapy causes serotonin release. Anti-emetics such as ondansetron can be prescribed.

Basic anatomy

Skull

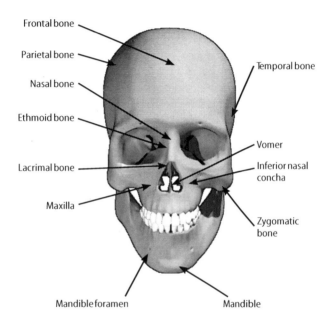

Frontal bone

Parietal bone

Nasal bone

Ethmoid bone

Lacrimal bone

Maxilla

Temporal bone

Vomer

Inferior nasal concha

Zygomatic bone

Mandible foramen

Mandible

Pelvis

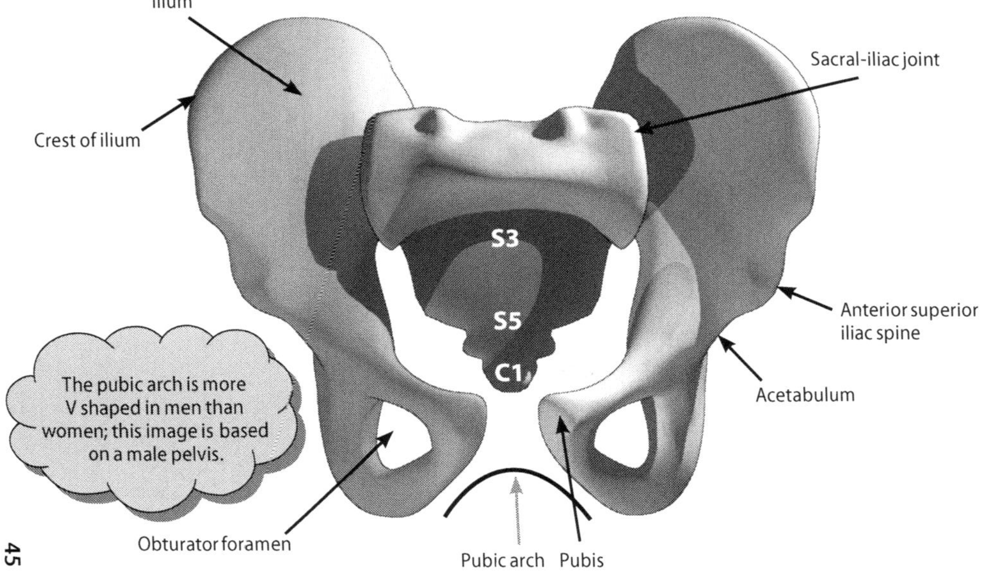

Sacral-iliac joint

Anterior superior iliac spine

Acetabulum

Pubic arch

Pubis

S3

S5

C1

Obturator foramen

Ilium

Crest of ilium

The pubic arch is more V shaped in men than women; this image is based on a male pelvis.

Vertebral levels

C1: Base of skull, hard palate

C3: Angle of mandible, hyoid bone, epiglottis

C4: Thyroid cartilage, thyroid upper level

C6: Cricoid cartilage, pharynx, isthmus of thyroid gland

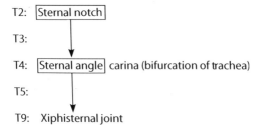

T2: Sternal notch

T3:

T4: Sternal angle carina (bifurcation of trachea)

T5:

T9: Xiphisternal joint

T10: Oesophagus enters diaphragm

T11: Oesophagus enters stomach

T12: Abdominal aorta

L1: Spinal cord, foramen magnum, renal arteries

L2: Gall bladder

L3: Umbilicus, lower costal margin

L4: Umbilicus, iliac crest, bifurcation of abdominal aorta

Larynx:	C3–C6
Trachea:	C6–T4
Oesophagus:	C6–T11 (22 cm long)
Aortic arch:	2.5 cm below suprasternal notch–T4
Stomach:	T4–T10
Spleen:	9th rib–11th rib
Right kidney:	T11–L3
Pancreas:	L1–2
Left kidney:	T11–L3
Pulmonary artery:	Arises at 2nd costal cartilage, Bifurcates at 3rd left costal cartilage
Liver:	5th costal space – 10th costal space
Rectum:	Line joining posterior superior iliac crest – S3
Pituitary gland:	2.5 cm Ant + 2.5 cm Sup to tragus
Parotid:	Extends from tragus – 2 cm below angle of mandible
Pineal gland:	3 cm Sup + 1.5 cm Post of tragus

Manual handling

Good manual handling is essential in order to prevent injury to yourself and others.

Bending your knees when lifting/putting down objects.	Having a stooped back when picking up heavy objects.
Keeping the heavy load close to your body.	Rushing and not asking for additional help with awkward/heavy loads.
Having a stable base at all times.	Bending and twisting at the same time.
Using a 'rocking' motion when assisting a patient to stand up, ensuring that they move to the edge of their seat first.	Allowing the patient to hold onto you in order to pull themselves up.
Not undertaking strain on your back unnecessarily.	Not clearing a pathway when moving a load or patient.
Using aids such as a pat-slide and a slide sheet.	Using equipment which has an out-of-date service check.
Keeping your head up when carrying loads.	Not applying the brakes to movable equipment, for example a wheelchair.

Infection control

Hand washing is important in order to prevent the spread of infection to staff and patients.
Some patients may be immunosuppressed due to chemotherapy treatments, therefore great care and attention should be given to hand hygiene.

> **WHEN SHOULD I WASH MY HANDS?**

1. Before touching the patient.

2. When leaving the treatment room in between beams.

3. After each time you touch the patient.

4. After any contact with bodily fluid (you should be wearing gloves for this too).

5. After the patient has had their treatment.

> **WHAT SHOULD I USE TO WASH MY HANDS?**

For the times you are in a hurry, for example when leaving the room to switch on, **alcohol gel** should be provided on the walls to quickly use on the way out. You shouldn't use this every time; in between patients **soap and warm water** is more appropriate. Do not use alcohol gel when your hands are visibly dirty.

On the walls by a sink there should be a poster instructing you on how to wash your hands most effectively.

Basic life support

In an emergency dial '2222' in order to call the crash team. Tell the operator if the patient is a child or an adult and if possible have the patient's notes at hand to help the crash team.

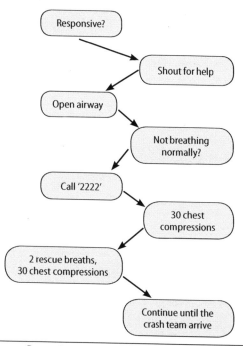

Reference: Resuscitation Council (2010) *Adult Basic Life Support*. Available at: www.resus.org.uk/pages/bls.pdf.

The recovery position

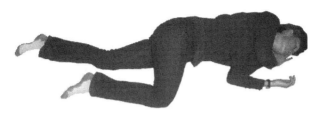

Points to remember

- Ensure the airway is open by keeping their head tilted back – adjusting their hand may help you with this.
- Check their breathing regularly.
- If the patient is still in the recovery position after 30 minutes, put them into the recovery position on their other side.
- NEVER put anything in their mouth.
- NEVER move the patient unless instructed to do so.

Reference: Barraclough, N. (2007) *First Aid Made Easy*. Dorchester: First on Scene Training Ltd, p. 11.

Medical terminology

Accelerated radiotherapy: the radiation dose is given over a shorter period of time than conventional treatment.

Acute toxicity: side-effects which occur immediately or shortly after treatment. In general these side-effects reduce over time.

Adenocarcinoma: cancer of a gland or glandular tissue, which arises in the epithelium.

Adenoma: a benign tumour.

Adjuvant treatment: treatment given in addition to the primary treatment to increase long-term survival.

Adverse effect: an unwanted side-effect of treatment.

Analgesic: drugs used to relieve pain.

Antiemetic drug: used to treat nausea and vomiting.

Asymptomatic: without symptoms.

Benign: non-cancerous tumours that do not invade or destroy local tissues and do not spread to other sites in the body.

Biopsy: a diagnostic test in which a small amount of tissue or cells are removed from the body for microscopic examination.

Carcinoma: any cancerous tumour arising from cells in the covering surface layer or lining membrane of an organ.

Carcinoma _in situ_: the earliest stage of a cancer in which it has not yet spread from the surface layer of cells of an organ.

Catheter: a flexible tube inserted into the body to drain or introduce fluids.

Combined modality therapy: a combination of two types of treatment, e.g. chemotherapy and radiotherapy.

Cystitis: inflammation of the bladder lining.

Dysphagia: difficulty swallowing.

Dysphasia: inability to select the words with which to speak and write.

Erythema: redness of the skin.

Fractionation: dividing the total dose of radiation into smaller doses conventionally given once a day, Monday to Friday.

Haematuria: blood in urine.

Haemoptysis: coughing up blood.

Hyperfractionation: increasing the number of fractions compared to conventional treatment. This decreases the dose per fraction.

Hypofractionation: decreasing the number of fractions compared to conventional treatment. This increases the dose per fraction.

Lumpectomy: surgical treatment for breast cancer in which only the cancer tissue is removed.

Malignant: cancerous tumour that spreads from its original location to form secondary tumour in other parts of the body.

Mastectomy: surgical removal of the entire breast.

Metastasis: a secondary tumour which has spread from a primary tumour in another part of the body.

Micturition: passing urine.

Mucus: thick slimy fluid secreted by mucous membranes.

Neoadjuvant: treatment given in addition to the primary treatment but administered prior to primary treatment.

Palliative treatment: treatment of any type that is intended to relieve the signs and symptoms of cancer and improve the patient's quality of life.

Proctitis: inflammation of the rectum.

Prostatectomy: an operation to remove part or all of the prostate gland.

Radical treatment: treatment of any type which is intended to cure the cancer.

Xerostomia: dryness of the mouth.

References: The British Medical Association (BMA) (2009) *Illustrated Medical Dictionary.* 2nd ed. London: Dorling Kindersley, p. 501.
McArdle, O. and O'Mahony, D. (2008) *Oncology.* London: Churchill Livingstone, pp. 119–120.

Notes